# Table Of Contents

## Introduction To The Mediterranean Diet

Thought to be the heart-healthiest of diets, the Mediterranean Diet is a style of eating popular among people who live along the Mediterranean Sea. A foundation of this diet is fish high in omega-3 fatty acid, which has been proven to reduce inflammation.

"The Mediterranean Diet has been shown to be anti-inflammatory because of its focus on whole foods and omega-3 fatty acids." According to nutritionists, "It also eliminates processed oils, like cottonseed and soybean oil, which are found in many ultra-processed foods."

In today's fast-paced world, where processed foods and sedentary lifestyles have become the norm, the prevalence of chronic inflammatory conditions is on the rise. While inflammation is a natural response that helps the body fight infections and heal injuries, chronic inflammation can lead to a range of health issues, including heart disease, diabetes, and autoimmune disorders. Fortunately, adopting an anti-inflammatory diet can be a powerful tool to combat inflammation and promote overall well-being. In this guide, we will delve into the science-backed benefits of an anti-inflammatory diet and explore key dietary choices that can nourish your body for optimal health.

### Understanding Inflammation and Chronic Disease

Inflammation is the body's natural defense mechanism against harmful stimuli, such as pathogens and injuries. It involves the activation of the immune system, leading to an increased flow of blood and immune cells to the affected area. However, when this response becomes prolonged or excessive, chronic inflammation can occur, triggering a cascade of detrimental effects on our health.

Chronic inflammation has been linked to various health conditions, including cardiovascular disease, obesity, arthritis, and gastrointestinal disorders. Lifestyle factors, such as poor diet choices, lack of exercise, and chronic stress, can contribute to this persistent inflammatory state.

The Role of an Anti-Inflammatory Diet

An anti-inflammatory diet focuses on consuming foods that can help reduce inflammation and support the body's natural healing processes. By emphasizing nutrient-rich, whole foods, this diet can have a profound impact on overall health and well-being.

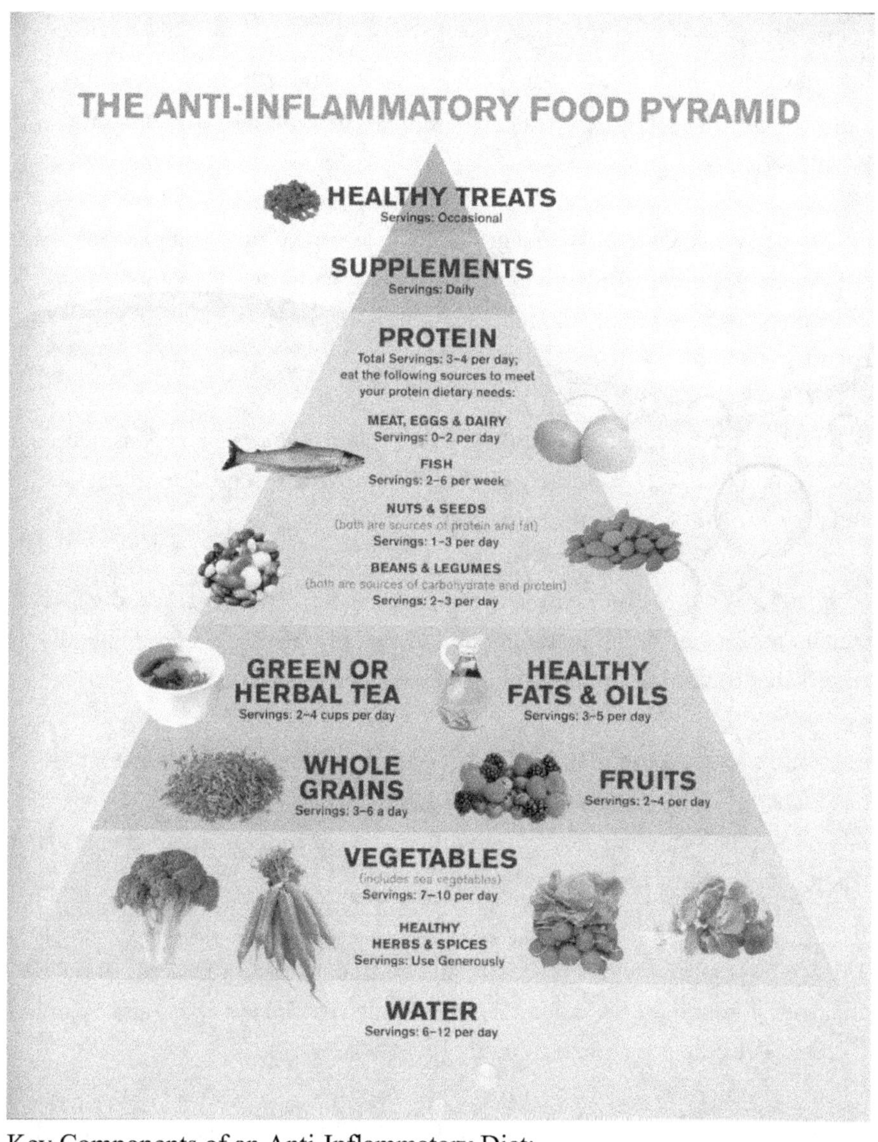


Key Components of an Anti-Inflammatory Diet:

1. Load Up on Fruits and Vegetables: Colorful fruits and vegetables are rich in antioxidants, vitamins, and minerals that combat oxidative stress and inflammation. Incorporate a diverse range of produce into your meals, such as leafy greens, berries, broccoli, and bell peppers, to reap their anti-inflammatory benefits.

2. Opt for Healthy Fats: Replace saturated and trans fats with heart-healthy fats, like those found in avocados, olive oil, nuts, and fatty fish. These fats contain omega-3 fatty acids, which are known for their anti-inflammatory properties.

3. Choose Whole Grains: Whole grains, such as brown rice, quinoa, and oats, are excellent sources of fiber and nutrients. They help stabilize blood sugar levels and promote gut health, reducing the risk of inflammation-related conditions.

4. Embrace Lean Protein: Incorporate lean protein sources, like beans, lentils, poultry, and tofu, into your diet. These foods provide essential amino acids and play a role in tissue repair and immune function.

5. Spice Up Your Meals: Certain spices, such as turmeric, ginger, and garlic, contain potent anti-inflammatory compounds. Sprinkle these spices liberally in your dishes to add flavor and health-boosting benefits.

6. Limit Processed Foods and Added Sugars: Processed foods often contain trans fats, refined sugars, and chemical additives that can promote inflammation. Minimize their consumption and opt for homemade meals using whole, unprocessed ingredients.

The Mediterranean diet is inspired by the traditional dietary patterns of countries bordering the Mediterranean Sea, such as Greece, Italy, and Spain. It emphasizes the consumption of:

1. Fruits and Vegetables: Plenty of fresh fruits and vegetables are central to the Mediterranean diet. These provide essential vitamins, minerals, and antioxidants.

2. Whole Grains: Whole grains like whole wheat, barley, quinoa, and oats are preferred over refined grains.

3. Healthy Fats: Olive oil is the primary source of fat in this diet, providing

monounsaturated fats that are beneficial for heart health. Nuts, seeds, and fatty fish (rich in omega-3 fatty acids) are also included.

4. Protein: Moderate consumption of fish, poultry, eggs, and dairy products is common. Red meat is consumed in smaller quantities.

5. Legumes: Beans, lentils, and chickpeas are staple sources of protein and fiber in the Mediterranean diet.

6. Dairy: Moderate consumption of yogurt and cheese is typical.

7. Red Wine (in moderation): Some Mediterranean diets include moderate consumption of red wine, which has been associated with certain health benefits. However, this aspect is optional and should be approached with moderation.

The anti-inflammatory diet focuses on foods that help reduce inflammation in the body, which is linked to various chronic diseases.

The diet includes:

1. Fruits and Vegetables: A wide variety of colorful fruits and vegetables, which are rich in antioxidants and anti-inflammatory compounds.

2. Healthy Fats: Emphasis on foods high in omega-3 fatty acids, such as fatty fish, walnuts, flaxseeds, and chia seeds.

3. Whole Grains: Whole grains that are minimally processed and high in fiber, like quinoa, brown rice, and whole wheat.

4. Lean Proteins: Fish, poultry, legumes, and plant-based proteins are preferred over red meat and processed meats.

5. Nuts and Seeds: These provide healthy fats and anti-inflammatory properties.

6. Herbs and Spices: Turmeric, ginger, garlic, and other herbs and spices with anti-inflammatory benefits are encouraged.

7. Limited Added Sugars and Processed Foods: Refined sugars and processed foods that may contribute to inflammation are minimized.

Both diets encourage reducing the intake of processed foods, sugary beverages, and unhealthy fats. They promote a balanced and whole-foods approach to eating, which can support overall health and well-being. In summary, while the Mediterranean diet and the anti-inflammatory diet share common principles and health-promoting aspects, the anti-inflammatory diet specifically emphasizes foods that can help reduce inflammation in the body. The Mediterranean diet, on the other hand, encompasses a broader cultural eating pattern with a focus on fresh and wholesome foods, including the benefits of olive oil and moderate wine consumption.

### Scale Back on Processed Foods

The first key to minimizing inflammation is cutting foods that cause it. An anti-inflammatory diet is one that includes minimally processed foods. That typically means staying away from anything that comes in a box or a bag, or anything that has a laundry list of ingredients — especially if they start with sugar, salt or a processed oil and include ingredients you don't recognize.

Examples include:

• Sweets, like commercial baked goods, pre-packaged desserts, ice cream and candy.
• Snack foods, like potato chips and microwave popcorn.
• Processed meats, including bacon, sausage, hot dogs, bologna, pepperoni and salami.
• Processed cheeses, like nacho cheese dip and American cheese slices.

• Sugary beverages, including soda and sports drinks.
• Fried foods, like fried chicken and French fries.

Even so-called healthy snacks like granola bars, trail mix and baked chips can have a lot of processed ingredients, including added sodium and sugar.

## Focus on Whole Foods

When you've cut out the processed stuff, what's left? Whole foods, of course! A whole food is a one-ingredient food, an entire entity: an apple, an orange, a cucumber.

In addition to fruits and vegetables, other examples include:
• Brown or wild rice.
• Chicken/turkey breast.
• Eggs.
• Fish (especially oily fish, such as salmon, tuna, herring or mackerel).
• Legumes, like dried beans and peas.
• Nuts and seeds.
• Oats.

In short, if you can find it in nature, it's probably a whole food. So do any processed foods make the grade? Foods that have more than one ingredient can still be made up of whole foods — for example, store-bought hummus, dried fruit and nut snack mix or a pasta sauce. The key is to always review the ingredient list. That means choosing breads and pastas that are minimally processed, minimally preserved and made with whole grains.

## Try a Diet Proven to Reduce Inflammation

Again, there's no one-size-fits-all anti-inflammatory diet. But two styles of eating have been shown to help: the Mediterranean Diet and the DASH Diet. "Positive research reports that these diets are successful in reducing inflammation, as well as cholesterol, weight, blood pressure and blood sugar."

The Mediterranean Diet

Thought to be the heart-healthiest of diets, the Mediterranean Diet is a style of eating popular among people who live along the Mediterranean Sea. A foundation of this diet is fish high in omega-3 fatty acid, which has been proven to reduce inflammation.

The Mediterranean Diet has been shown to be anti-inflammatory because of its focus on whole foods and omega-3 fatty acids. It also eliminates processed oils, like cottonseed and soybean oil, which are found in many ultra-processed foods.

The DASH diet

DASH, which stands for Dietary Approaches to Stop Hypertension, is a diet designed to reduce high blood pressure. This diet has been shown to reduce inflammation, probably because it reduces blood pressure and promotes weight loss. Remember, both high blood pressure and obesity are associated with inflammation.

Like the Mediterranean Diet, the DASH Diet focuses on whole foods and limits protein, sweets and processed foods. But DASH includes a bit more dairy, and it doesn't specifically encourage fish or extra-virgin olive oil.

Is vegetarianism anti-inflammatory? Though meat can be inflammatory, keep in mind that cutting animal products doesn't necessarily mean eating healthfully. Eating a plant-based diet can help suppress inflammation, but vegetarian, pescetarian and even vegan diets can still include foods like potato chips, fries and cookies.

To see anti-inflammatory benefits, you have to stick to whole foods.

If needed, try an elimination diet.

If you've cut out processed foods but still experience symptoms of inflammation, you may need to go a step further.

Finding the right anti-inflammatory diet for you is a matter of personalization and finding the foods that trigger your inflammation.

The best way to start is by trying an elimination diet and slowly cutting out potential trigger foods one by one.

Food sensitivity tests can help identify which foods increase your body's antibody response, too, which may be helpful if you can't seem to determine a culprit on your own.

How long does it take to see results? Starting an anti-inflammatory diet isn't a magic pill. Your results will vary based on the severity of your intolerance and inflammation. Drastic changes never lead to long-term success, so give yourself three to six months to make diet changes and to begin to see results.

Begin by making small changes that you know will be impactful, and then slowly continue to add on. In some cases, if you significantly react to a certain food, you may see results as soon as two to three weeks after eliminating that food from your diet. This can be very encouraging and motivating. People often will say that they never realized how bad they felt until they changed their diet and began to feel so much better.

There are a lot of different ways your body can react to an anti-inflammatory diet, they include:

• Clearer skin
• Decreased muscle or joint pain
• Decreased swelling in your hands and feet
• Fewer headache
• Improved gastrointestinal symptoms (diarrhea, gas, nausea, stomach pain)
• Improved sleep

- Less anxiety, stress and/or brain fog
- Less bloating
- Lower blood pressure
- Lower blood sugar
- More energy
- Weight loss.

**Supplements That Research Shows May Help Reduce Inflammation**

Curcumin is a compound found in the spice turmeric, which is commonly used in Indian cuisine and known for its bright yellow hue. It provides several impressive health benefits. Curcumin may help decrease inflammation in diabetes, heart disease, inflammatory bowel disease, and cancer, among other conditions. Curcumin is a natural compound found in turmeric, a yellow spice commonly used in Indian cuisine and traditional medicine. It has gained significant attention in recent years due to its potential health benefits. While curcumin's benefits are widely studied, it's essential to note that more research is needed to fully understand its effects on various health conditions. Some of the potential benefits of curcumin include:

1. Powerful Anti-Inflammatory Properties: Curcumin is known for its potent anti-inflammatory effects. It can help reduce inflammation by inhibiting certain enzymes and molecules responsible for the inflammatory response. This makes it potentially beneficial for conditions related to chronic inflammation, such as arthritis and inflammatory bowel disease.

2. Antioxidant Action: Curcumin is a powerful antioxidant that can neutralize harmful free radicals in the body. By doing so, it helps protect cells from oxidative damage, which is associated with aging and various chronic diseases.

3. Support for Joint Health: Due to its anti-inflammatory properties, curcumin may aid in alleviating joint pain and improving joint

flexibility in individuals with conditions like osteoarthritis or rheumatoid arthritis.

4. Potential Cardiovascular Benefits: Studies suggest that curcumin may have positive effects on heart health by improving endothelial function, reducing LDL cholesterol levels, and inhibiting platelet aggregation, which can help lower the risk of heart disease.

5. Cognitive Health Support: Some research indicates that curcumin may have neuroprotective effects, potentially benefiting brain health. It may help promote memory and cognitive function and could be beneficial in the prevention or management of neurodegenerative diseases like Alzheimer's.

6. Mood and Emotional Well-being: Curcumin may have a positive impact on mood and emotional well-being. Some studies have shown that it can potentially alleviate symptoms of depression and anxiety.

7. Potential Anti-Cancer Properties: While research is still ongoing, some studies suggest that curcumin may have anti-cancer properties. It has shown potential in inhibiting cancer cell growth, reducing tumor size, and preventing the spread of cancer cells.

8. Digestive Health Support: Curcumin's anti-inflammatory properties may benefit gastrointestinal health by reducing inflammation in conditions like ulcerative colitis and improving overall digestive function.

It's important to note that the bioavailability of curcumin is relatively low, meaning that the body absorbs and utilizes only a small portion of the curcumin consumed. To enhance its absorption, it is often recommended to consume curcumin with black pepper (piperine) or in liposomal or nanoparticle forms.

Fish oil supplements contain omega-3 fatty acids, which are vital for good health. They may help decrease the inflammation associated with diabetes, heart disease, and other conditions. The two primary omega-3s in fish oil are eicosapentaenoic acid (EPA) and docosahexaenoic acid (DHA). Your body converts them to ALA, which is an essential fatty acid (17Trusted Source). DHA, in particular, has been shown to have anti-inflammatory effects that reduce cytokine levels and promote gut health. It may also decrease the inflammation and muscle damage that occur after exercise, but more research is needed. Fish oil is a popular dietary supplement that is rich in omega-3 fatty acids, particularly eicosapentaenoic acid (EPA) and docosahexaenoic acid (DHA). These essential fatty acids offer numerous health benefits, making fish oil a widely recommended supplement.

Here are some of the key benefits of fish oil:

1. Heart Health: Omega-3 fatty acids in fish oil have been shown to support heart health by reducing triglyceride levels, decreasing blood pressure, and improving overall cholesterol profiles. They can also help prevent the formation of harmful blood clots and inflammation in blood vessels, reducing the risk of heart disease.

2. Brain Health: DHA, a major component of fish oil, is essential for brain development and function. Consuming sufficient omega-3 fatty acids has been linked to better cognitive function, memory, and mood regulation. Some studies suggest that regular fish oil intake may help reduce the risk of neurodegenerative diseases like Alzheimer's.

3. Joint Health: Fish oil's anti-inflammatory properties may benefit individuals with joint conditions, such as rheumatoid arthritis and osteoarthritis. Omega-3s can help reduce joint pain, stiffness, and inflammation, enhancing joint mobility and overall comfort.

4. Eye Health: DHA is also a crucial component of the retina in the eye. Consuming fish oil may support eye health, reducing the risk of age-related macular degeneration and dry eye syndrome.

5. Skin Health: The anti-inflammatory properties of fish oil can help improve skin health by reducing inflammation associated with skin conditions like psoriasis and eczema. Additionally, omega-3 fatty acids can promote skin hydration and elasticity, contributing to a more radiant complexion.

6. Immune System Support: Omega-3 fatty acids play a role in supporting a healthy immune system. They can enhance immune function, help fight off infections, and reduce chronic inflammation, which is beneficial for overall immune health.

7. Pregnancy and Infant Development: Omega-3 fatty acids are crucial during pregnancy for fetal brain and eye development. Pregnant women who consume fish oil may support their baby's cognitive development and reduce the risk of preterm birth.

8. Weight Management: Fish oil supplements, when combined with a healthy diet and exercise, may aid in weight loss efforts. They can increase feelings of fullness, improve metabolism, and reduce fat storage. It's important to note that while fish oil offers numerous benefits, it should not be used as a replacement for a balanced diet.

Consuming fatty fish like salmon, mackerel, and sardines, along with a variety of plant-based omega-3 sources, is also recommended for a comprehensive approach to health and well-being.

Ginger root is commonly used in cooking and has a history of use in herbal medicine too. It's also used as a home remedy to treat indigestion and nausea, including morning sickness during pregnancy. Two components of ginger, gingerol and zingerone, may help reduce inflammation related to several health conditions, including type 2 diabetes. Ginger consumption may also positively impact HbA1c (blood sugar control over 3 months) over time. Ginger is a popular spice known for its unique flavor and aroma, but it also boasts a wide range of health benefits. For centuries, ginger has been used in traditional medicine and culinary practices around the world. Here are some of the key benefits of ginger:

1. Digestive Aid: Ginger is renowned for its ability to alleviate digestive discomfort. It can help reduce bloating, gas, and indigestion by promoting the smooth movement of food through the digestive system. Ginger is also effective in relieving nausea, making it a natural remedy for motion sickness and morning sickness during pregnancy.

2. Anti-Inflammatory Properties: Ginger contains bioactive compounds with potent anti-inflammatory effects. Regular consumption of ginger can help reduce inflammation in the body, which may contribute to alleviating symptoms of inflammatory conditions like osteoarthritis and rheumatoid arthritis.

3. Immune System Support: The immune-boosting properties of ginger can help strengthen the body's defenses against infections and illnesses. It contains antioxidants that combat free radicals and oxidative stress, supporting overall immune health.

4. Pain Relief: The anti-inflammatory effects of ginger also make it beneficial for pain relief. It may help reduce muscle soreness, menstrual pain, and headaches when consumed regularly.

5. Cardiovascular Health: Ginger has been shown to support cardiovascular health by helping to lower blood pressure and improve blood circulation. It may also help reduce cholesterol levels, lowering the risk of heart disease.

6. Anti-Nausea and Morning Sickness: Ginger is well-known for its ability to alleviate nausea and vomiting, making it a popular remedy for pregnancy-related morning sickness and chemotherapy-induced nausea.

7. Respiratory Health: Ginger's warming properties can be soothing for respiratory issues such as coughs and sore throats. It may help ease congestion and promote better respiratory function.

8. Weight Management: Consuming ginger may aid in weight management efforts by boosting metabolism and promoting feelings of fullness, which can help control appetite and reduce overeating.

9. Antimicrobial Effects: Ginger has natural antimicrobial properties that can help combat certain types of bacteria and viruses, potentially reducing the risk of infections.

10. Skin Health: The anti-inflammatory and antioxidant properties of ginger can contribute to improved skin health by reducing skin redness, irritation, and signs of aging.

Ginger can be enjoyed in various forms, including fresh, dried, powdered, and as a supplement. Incorporating ginger into your diet can be as simple as adding it to teas, soups, stir-fries, smoothies, and various culinary dishes.

Resveratrol is an antioxidant found in grapes, blueberries, and other fruits with purple skin. It's also found in red wine, dark chocolate, and peanuts. It's been widely studied for its anti-inflammatory potential in people with chronic conditions like liver disease, obesity, and ulcerative colitis (UC), as well as in people without chronic conditions. Resveratrol is a natural polyphenol compound found in certain plants, fruits, and red wine. It has gained significant attention for its potential health benefits. Here are some of the key benefits of resveratrol:

1. Antioxidant Properties: Resveratrol is a powerful antioxidant that helps neutralize harmful free radicals in the body. By doing so, it helps protect cells from oxidative damage, which is associated with aging and various chronic diseases.

2. Heart Health: Resveratrol has been linked to improved heart health. It may help reduce LDL cholesterol levels (the "bad" cholesterol) and prevent the oxidation of LDL cholesterol, which can

lower the risk of heart disease. Additionally, resveratrol may promote healthy blood flow and support cardiovascular function.

3. Anti-Inflammatory Effects: Resveratrol has anti-inflammatory properties that may help reduce inflammation in the body. Chronic inflammation is associated with various health conditions, including heart disease, diabetes, and certain cancers.

4. Brain Health: Resveratrol has shown promise in supporting brain health and cognitive function. Some studies suggest that it may help protect against neurodegenerative diseases like Alzheimer's and Parkinson's by reducing oxidative stress and inflammation in the brain.

5. Anti-Cancer Potential: Research indicates that resveratrol may have anti-cancer properties. It has shown potential in inhibiting the growth of cancer cells and preventing tumor formation. However, more research is needed to fully understand its effects on different types of cancer.

6. Blood Sugar Regulation: Resveratrol may help improve insulin sensitivity and regulate blood sugar levels, making it potentially beneficial for individuals with type 2 diabetes or those at risk of developing diabetes.

7. Skin Health: Resveratrol's antioxidant and anti-inflammatory properties can benefit the skin by protecting against UV-induced skin damage, reducing signs of aging, and promoting a more youthful appearance.

8. Weight Management: Some studies suggest that resveratrol may have positive effects on weight management. It may help reduce fat accumulation, improve metabolism, and support healthy weight loss efforts.

It's important to note that while resveratrol shows promising health benefits in research studies, more extensive human trials are needed to fully establish its efficacy and safety. Additionally, the amount of resveratrol naturally found in foods like red grapes and berries is relatively low, so consuming these foods alone may not provide sufficient levels for significant health effects.

Spirulina is a type of blue-green algae with strong antioxidant effects. Studies have shown that it reduces inflammation, promotes healthy aging, and may strengthen the immune system. Although most research has investigated spirulina's effects on animals, studies in older adults have shown that it may improve inflammatory markers, anemia, and immune function. Spirulina is a type of blue-green algae that is often referred to as a "superfood" due to its dense nutritional content. It has been consumed for centuries and is now widely available as a dietary supplement.

Here are some of the key benefits of spirulina:

1. Rich Source of Nutrients: Spirulina is packed with essential nutrients, including protein, vitamins (such as B vitamins and vitamin K), minerals (like iron, calcium, and magnesium), and antioxidants. It is especially valued as a plant-based protein source, making it an excellent option for vegans and vegetarians.

2. Powerful Antioxidant Properties: Spirulina contains a variety of antioxidants, such as phycocyanin, which helps protect cells from oxidative damage caused by free radicals. These antioxidants may contribute to overall health and reduce the risk of chronic diseases.

3. Supports Immune Function: Spirulina has immune-boosting properties that can enhance the body's defense against infections and illnesses. The combination of antioxidants and immune-supporting nutrients helps strengthen the immune system.

4. Anti-Inflammatory Effects: Spirulina has demonstrated anti-inflammatory properties, which may help reduce inflammation in the body. Chronic inflammation is associated with various health

conditions, and incorporating spirulina into the diet may offer some relief.

5. Cardiovascular Health: Studies suggest that spirulina may have beneficial effects on heart health by reducing LDL cholesterol levels and triglycerides, and improving the ratio of HDL (good) to LDL (bad) cholesterol. These effects may contribute to a decreased risk of heart disease.

6. Supports Detoxification: Spirulina is believed to aid in detoxifying the body by assisting in the elimination of heavy metals and other toxins. Its high chlorophyll content is thought to be responsible for this detoxifying effect.

7. Promotes Healthy Gut: Spirulina has prebiotic properties, which means it can help support the growth of beneficial gut bacteria. A healthy gut microbiome is essential for digestion, nutrient absorption, and overall gut health.

8. Energy and Endurance: Due to its rich nutrient content, spirulina is often used as a natural energy booster and to improve endurance during physical activities. 9. Potential Anti-Cancer Effects: Some studies suggest that spirulina may have anti-cancer properties, attributed to its antioxidant and immune-enhancing effects. However, more research is needed to fully understand its impact on cancer prevention and treatment.

Vitamin D is an essential fat-soluble nutrient that plays a key role in immune health and may have some powerful anti-inflammatory properties. In several studies, researchers have noted a link between low vitamin D levels and the presence of inflammation. Vitamin D is a crucial nutrient that plays various essential roles in the body. It is often referred to as the "sunshine vitamin" because the skin can synthesize it when exposed to sunlight.

Here are some of the key benefits of vitamin D:

1. Bone Health: Vitamin D is essential for the proper absorption of calcium and phosphorus, which are vital minerals for maintaining strong and healthy bones. It helps regulate calcium levels in the blood, ensuring that there is enough calcium available to support bone formation and maintenance.

2. Immune System Support: Vitamin D plays a significant role in supporting the immune system. It helps activate immune cells and enhances the body's defense against infections and diseases.

3. Mood and Mental Health: Some studies suggest that vitamin D may have a positive impact on mood and mental health. Adequate vitamin D levels have been linked to a reduced risk of depression and other mood disorders.

4. Cardiovascular Health: Research indicates that vitamin D may help reduce the risk of cardiovascular diseases by supporting heart health. It may help lower blood pressure, improve blood vessel function, and reduce inflammation in the cardiovascular system.

5. Cancer Prevention: Some studies suggest that maintaining sufficient vitamin D levels may be associated with a reduced risk of certain cancers, including breast, prostate, and colorectal cancers. However, more research is needed to fully understand this relationship.

6. Weight Management: Adequate vitamin D levels may play a role in weight management. Some research suggests that higher vitamin D levels are associated with lower body fat and a reduced risk of obesity.

7. Muscle Function: Vitamin D is involved in muscle function and may help improve muscle strength and performance, especially in older adults.

8. Diabetes Prevention: Some studies suggest that maintaining adequate vitamin D levels may reduce the risk of developing type 2

diabetes.

9. Skin Health: While vitamin D synthesis primarily occurs in the skin, the nutrient also supports overall skin health. It may help reduce inflammation and improve certain skin conditions like psoriasis.

It's important to note that vitamin D deficiency can lead to health problems, including bone disorders like rickets in children and osteomalacia in adults. Severe deficiency may result in a condition called osteoporosis, characterized by weak and brittle bones. Vitamin D can be obtained through exposure to sunlight, dietary sources (such as fatty fish, fortified foods, and certain mushrooms), and supplements. It's crucial to maintain adequate vitamin D levels through a balanced diet and, if necessary, under the guidance of a healthcare professional.

Bromelain is a powerful enzyme found in pineapple that gives the fruit its astringency. Bromelain in the reason pineapple leaves a burning sensation if you eat too much. However, it also has some potential anti-inflammatory properties. In fact, bromelain has the same anti-inflammatory capacity as nonsteroidal anti-inflammatory drugs (NSAIDs), but with the bonus of fewer side effects. Bromelain is a group of enzymes derived from the pineapple plant (Ananas comosus). It has been used for centuries in traditional medicine practices, and modern research has identified several potential health benefits associated with bromelain.

Here are some of the key benefits:

1. Digestive Aid: Bromelain is known for its digestive properties. It helps break down proteins in the digestive tract, improving digestion and nutrient absorption. Due to its digestive benefits, bromelain is often used to alleviate digestive issues like bloating, gas, and

indigestion.

2. Anti-Inflammatory Effects: Bromelain has potent anti-inflammatory properties, making it useful in reducing inflammation and swelling associated with injuries, surgical procedures, and inflammatory conditions like osteoarthritis and sinusitis.

3. Immune System Support: Bromelain may help support the immune system by enhancing the activity of immune cells and promoting a healthy immune response. It can help the body defend against infections and illnesses.

4. Sinus Relief: Due to its anti-inflammatory properties, bromelain is often used as a natural remedy to alleviate sinusitis symptoms. It can help reduce nasal inflammation and congestion, making it easier to breathe.

5. Sports Injuries and Muscle Recovery: Some studies suggest that bromelain may aid in reducing pain, swelling, and bruising associated with sports injuries and muscle strains. It is sometimes used to support muscle recovery after intense physical activity.

6. Respiratory Health: Bromelain's anti-inflammatory effects may benefit respiratory health by reducing inflammation in the airways. It may help alleviate symptoms of respiratory conditions like asthma and bronchitis.

7. Blood Clot Prevention: Some research indicates that bromelain may have blood-thinning properties, which can help prevent the formation of blood clots. However, individuals taking blood-thinning medications should use bromelain with caution and under the supervision of a healthcare professional.

8. Skin Health: Bromelain's anti-inflammatory and exfoliating properties make it a popular ingredient in skincare products. It can help reduce redness, swelling, and improve skin texture.

9. Cancer Treatment Support: While more research is needed, some studies suggest that bromelain may have potential as an adjuvant

therapy for cancer treatment. It may enhance the effectiveness of certain chemotherapy drugs and radiation therapy.

Bromelain is available in supplement form and can also be obtained by consuming fresh pineapple or drinking pineapple juice. However, bromelain supplements are more concentrated and standardized for specific purposes.

Green tea has long been used in traditional medicine, and it's rich in compounds that may provide many health benefits, such as epigallocatechin-3-gallate (EGCG), caffeine, and chlorogenic acid. One potential benefit is that it's extremely anti-inflammatory. Green tea extract is derived from the leaves of the Camellia sinensis plant, the same plant used to make green tea. It is a concentrated form of the beneficial compounds found in green tea.

Here are some of the key benefits of green tea extract:
1. Powerful Antioxidant: Green tea extract is rich in antioxidants, particularly catechins, which help neutralize free radicals and protect the body from oxidative stress. This antioxidant activity can reduce cellular damage and lower the risk of chronic diseases.
2. Weight Management: Some studies suggest that green tea extract may aid in weight management by boosting metabolism and increasing fat oxidation. It can help the body burn more calories and fat, potentially supporting weight loss efforts.
3. Heart Health: Green tea extract has been shown to have positive effects on cardiovascular health. It may help lower LDL cholesterol levels, reduce blood pressure, and improve overall heart function.
4. Brain Health: The antioxidants in green tea extract may have neuroprotective effects, supporting brain health and reducing the risk of cognitive decline. Some studies suggest that green tea extract may

help improve memory and cognitive function.

5. Liver Health: Green tea extract may benefit liver health by protecting the liver from damage caused by toxins and promoting its detoxification processes.

6. Immune System Support: The catechins in green tea extract can enhance the function of the immune system, helping the body defend against infections and illnesses.

7. Anti-Inflammatory Effects: Green tea extract has anti-inflammatory properties that can help reduce inflammation in the body, potentially benefiting individuals with inflammatory conditions.

8. Skin Health: The antioxidants in green tea extract can help protect the skin from UV damage, reduce redness and irritation, and promote a more youthful appearance.

9. Oral Health: Green tea extract may have a positive impact on oral health. It can help inhibit the growth of bacteria in the mouth, reducing the risk of cavities and gum disease.

10. Cancer Prevention: Some studies suggest that the antioxidants in green tea extract may have anticancer properties. They may help inhibit the growth of cancer cells and reduce the risk of certain types of cancer, such as breast, prostate, and colorectal cancer. However, more research is needed in this area.

It's important to note that while green tea extract offers potential health benefits, it should not be considered a substitute for a balanced diet and a healthy lifestyle. Additionally, green tea extract supplements may contain caffeine, which can cause adverse effects in some individuals, such as insomnia or jitteriness.

Garlic, like ginger, pineapple, and fatty fish, is a common food that's rich in anti-inflammatory compounds. Garlic is especially high in a compound called allicin, a potent anti-inflammatory agent that may also help strengthen the immune system to better ward off disease-causing pathogens. Garlic (Allium sativum) is a widely used herb known for its distinct flavor and aroma. It has been used for both culinary and medicinal purposes for thousands of years.

Here are some of the key benefits of garlic:

1. Cardiovascular Health: Garlic is known for its potential to support heart health. It can help lower LDL cholesterol levels (the "bad" cholesterol) and reduce blood pressure, which may lower the risk of heart disease and stroke.

2. Immune System Support: Garlic has immune-boosting properties due to its active compounds, including allicin. Regular consumption of garlic may help strengthen the immune system and increase the body's ability to fight off infections and illnesses.

3. Antioxidant Properties: Garlic contains antioxidants that help neutralize free radicals in the body, reducing oxidative stress and supporting overall health.

4. Anti-Inflammatory Effects: The compounds in garlic, such as allicin and sulfur-containing compounds, have anti-inflammatory properties that may help reduce inflammation in the body.

5. Cancer Prevention: Some studies suggest that garlic consumption may be associated with a reduced risk of certain types of cancer, particularly cancers of the digestive system, including the stomach and colon.

6. Improved Blood Circulation: Garlic has been found to have a mild blood-thinning effect, which can improve blood circulation and reduce the risk of blood clots.

7. Detoxification: Garlic may support the body's detoxification processes, helping to eliminate toxins and heavy metals from the body.

8. Respiratory Health: Garlic's anti-inflammatory and antimicrobial

properties can benefit respiratory health by helping to alleviate symptoms of common respiratory conditions like colds and flu.

9. Digestive Health: Garlic can aid in digestion by promoting the production of digestive enzymes and supporting a healthy gut microbiome.

10. Skin Health: The antimicrobial properties of garlic may help in treating skin conditions like acne and fungal infections.

It's important to note that while garlic offers numerous health benefits, it is not a substitute for medical treatment. It is most effective when incorporated as part of a balanced diet and a healthy lifestyle. Additionally, excessive garlic consumption may cause digestive discomfort and bad breath in some individuals.

Vitamin C, like vitamin D, is an essential vitamin that plays a huge role in immunity and inflammation. It's a powerful antioxidant, so it can reduce inflammation by neutralizing free radicals that cause oxidative damage to your cells (55Trusted Source). It also helps optimize the immune system in several other ways, which can help regulate inflammation — because inflammation is an immune response (55Trusted Source). In addition, high doses are commonly given intravenously to hospitalized patients with severe respiratory illnesses — like influenza, pneumonia, and even COVID-19 — to help reduce inflammation (56Trusted Source). In healthy people, though, doses higher than 2,000 mg may lead to diarrhea. Other than that, vitamin C supplements are safe and relatively symptom-free (57Trusted Source). However, it's also easy to meet your vitamin C needs through diet alone — green, red, orange, and yellow fruits and vegetables are all rich sources. Vitamin C, also known as ascorbic acid, is a water-soluble vitamin that plays a crucial role in various bodily functions.

Here are some of the key benefits of vitamin C:

1. Immune System Support: Vitamin C is well-known for its immune-boosting properties. It enhances the function of immune cells, such as white blood cells, which help the body fight off infections and illnesses.

2. Antioxidant Action: Vitamin C is a potent antioxidant that helps protect cells from oxidative damage caused by free radicals. This antioxidant activity contributes to overall health and may reduce the risk of chronic diseases.

3. Collagen Production: Vitamin C is essential for the synthesis of collagen, a protein that plays a vital role in maintaining healthy skin, joints, bones, and blood vessels. It supports wound healing and tissue repair.

4. Cardiovascular Health: Vitamin C has been associated with a reduced risk of heart disease. It may help lower blood pressure, improve blood vessel function, and reduce the risk of heart-related events.

5. Enhanced Iron Absorption: Vitamin C enhances the absorption of non-heme iron from plant-based foods, such as leafy greens and legumes. Consuming vitamin C-rich foods with iron-containing foods can help improve iron absorption and prevent iron deficiency anemia. 6. Skin Health: As an antioxidant, vitamin C helps protect the skin from sun damage and promotes a more youthful appearance by reducing the signs of aging, such as wrinkles and fine lines.

7. Eye Health: Vitamin C is beneficial for eye health. It helps protect against age-related macular degeneration (AMD) and may reduce the risk of cataracts.

8. Antihistamine Effects: Vitamin C has mild antihistamine properties, which may help alleviate symptoms of allergies and reduce histamine release

. 9. Brain Health: Some studies suggest that vitamin C may play a role in maintaining cognitive function and reducing the risk of neurodegenerative diseases like Alzheimer's.

10. Stress Reduction: Vitamin C can help reduce the levels of cortisol, a stress hormone, in the body, leading to a sense of relaxation and improved mood.

Vitamin C is essential for overall health and well-being, but the body cannot produce it on its own. Therefore, it's crucial to obtain sufficient vitamin C through diet o supplements.

Good dietary sources of vitamin C include citrus fruits (oranges, lemons, grapefruits), strawberries, kiwi, bell peppers, broccoli, and spinach.

As with any supplement, it's best to consult with a healthcare professional before starting fish oil supplementation, especially if you have any existing health conditions or are taking other medications. They can provide personalized advice and guidance based on your specific health needs.

### <u>Sample Menus</u>

Monday
• Breakfast: Greek yogurt with strawberries and chia seeds
• Lunch: a whole grain sandwich with hummus and vegetables
• Dinner: a tuna salad with greens and olive oil, as well as a fruit salad

Tuesday
• Breakfast: oatmeal with blueberries
• Lunch: caprese zucchini noodles with mozzarella, cherry tomatoes, olive oil, and balsamic vinegar
• Dinner: a salad with tomatoes, olives, cucumbers, farro, baked trout, and feta cheese

Wednesday
• Breakfast: an omelet with mushrooms, tomatoes, and onions
• Lunch: a whole grain sandwich with cheese and fresh vegetables
• Dinner: Mediterranean lasagna

Thursday
• Breakfast: yogurt with sliced fruit and nuts
• Lunch: a quinoa salad with chickpeas
• Dinner: broiled salmon with brown rice and vegetables

Friday
• Breakfast: eggs and sautéed vegetables with whole wheat toast
• Lunch: stuffed zucchini boats with pesto, turkey sausage, tomatoes, bell peppers, and cheese
• Dinner: grilled lamb with salad and baked potato

Saturday
• Breakfast: oatmeal with nuts and raisins or apple slices
• Lunch: lentil salad with feta, tomatoes, cucumbers, and olives
• Dinner: Mediterranean pizza made with whole wheat pita bread and topped with cheese, vegetables, and olives

Sunday
• Breakfast: an omelet with veggies and olives
• Lunch: falafel bowl with feta, onions, tomatoes, hummus, and rice
• Dinner: grilled chicken with vegetables, sweet potato fries, and fresh fruit

There's usually no need to count calories or track macronutrients (protein, fat, and carbs) on the Mediterranean diet, unless you are managing your glucose levels. But, it is essential to consume all food in moderation.

## **Healthy Snacks**

If you start feeling hungry between meals, there are plenty of healthy snack options, such as:
• a handful of nuts
• a piece of fruit
• baby carrots with hummus
• mixed berries
• grapes
• Greek yogurt • hard-boiled egg with salt and pepper
• apple slices with almond butter
• sliced bell peppers with guacamole
• cottage cheese with fresh fruit
• chia pudding

Eating out Many restaurants serve foods that fit in with the Mediterranean diet. Here are some tips to help adapt dishes when you're eating out:
1. Choose fish or seafood as your main dish.
2. Ask for grilled foods rather than fried, where possible.
3. Ask the server if your food can be cooked in extra virgin olive oil.
4. Choose whole grain bread, with olive oil instead of butter.
5. Add vegetables to your order.

### Shopping List

When shopping, opt for nutrient-dense foods, such as fruits, vegetables, nuts, seeds, legumes, and whole grains. Here are some basic Mediterranean diet items to add to your shopping list:
• Vegetables: carrots, onions, broccoli, spinach, kale, garlic, zucchini, mushrooms
• Frozen veggies: peas, carrots, broccoli, mixed vegetables
• Tubers: potatoes, sweet potatoes, yams
• Fruits: apples, bananas, oranges, grapes, melons, peaches, pears, strawberries, blueberries
• Grains: whole grain bread, whole grain pasta, quinoa, brown rice, oats
• Legumes: lentils, chickpeas, black beans, kidney beans
• Nuts: almonds, walnuts, cashews, pistachios, macadamia nuts

• Seeds: sunflower seeds, pumpkin seeds, chia seeds, hemp seeds
• Condiments: sea salt, pepper, turmeric, cinnamon, cayenne pepper, oregano
• Seafood: salmon, sardines, mackerel, trout, shrimp, mussels
• Dairy products: Greek yogurt, yogurt, milk
• Poultry: chicken, duck, turkey
• Eggs: chicken, quail, and duck eggs
• Healthy fats: extra virgin olive oil, olives, avocados, avocado oil

# If You Have Any Existing Health Conditions Or Are Taking Medications, It's A Good Idea To Consult With A Healthcare Professional Before Using Any Supplements Or Significantly Increasing Your Supplement Intake, As It May Interact With Certain Medications Or Medical Conditions. As With Any Dietary Supplement Or Natural Remedy, Moderation And Individual Tolerance Are Key Factors To Consider.